The Cheap Mediterranean Delicacies Cookbook

Tasty Recipes Affordable For Busy People and Beginners

Alison Russell

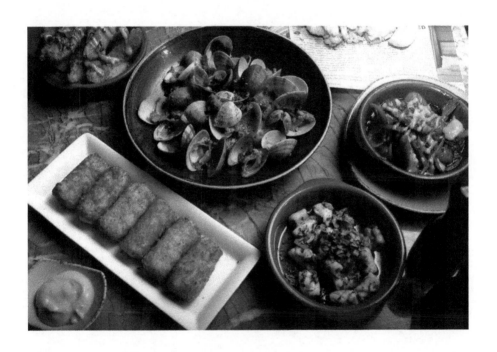

Table of contents

Breakfast

Poached Eggs with Avocado Purée

Preparation Time: 10 minutes

Cooking Time: 5 minutes

Servings: 4

Ingredients:

- 2 avocados, peeled and pitted
- 1/4 cup chopped fresh basil leaves
- 3 tablespoons red wine vinegar, divided
- Juice of 1 lemon
- Zest of 1 lemon
- 1 garlic clove, minced
- 1 teaspoon sea salt, divided
- 1/8 teaspoon freshly ground black pepper
- Pinch cayenne pepper, plus more as needed
- 4 eggs

Directions:

1. In a blender, combine the avocados, basil, 2 tablespoons of vinegar, the lemon juice and zest, garlic, 1/2 teaspoon of sea salt, pepper, and cayenne. Purée for about 1 minute until smooth.

2. Fill a 12-inch nonstick skillet about three-fourths full of water and place it over medium heat. Attach the remaining tablespoon of vinegar and the remaining 1/2 teaspoon of sea salt. Bring the water to a simmer.

3. Carefully crack the eggs into custard cups. Holding the cups just barely above the water, carefully slip the eggs into the simmering water, one at a time. Let the eggs sit for 5 minutes without agitating the pan or removing the lid.

4. Using a slotted spoon, carefully lift the eggs from the water, allowing them to drain completely. Place each egg on a plate and spoon the avocado purée over the top.

Nutrition:

Calories: 213, Protein: 2g, Total Carbohydrates: 11g, Fiber: 7g, Total Fat: 20g, Sodium: 475mg

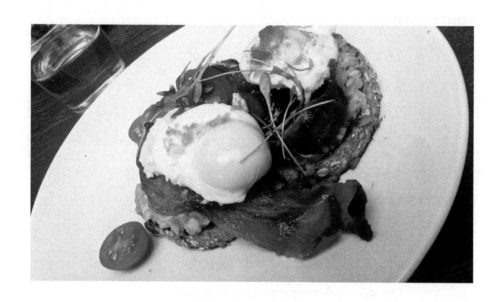

Sweet Potatoes with Coconut Flakes

Preparation Time: 15 minutes

Cooking Time: 1 hour

Servings: 2

Ingredients:

- 16 oz... sweet potatoes
- 1 tbsp.... maple syrup
- 1/4 c. Fat-free coconut Greek yogurt
- 1/8 c. unsweetened toasted coconut flakes
- 1 chopped apple

Directions:

1. Preheat oven to 400 0F.
2. Place your potatoes on a baking sheet. Bake them for 45 - 60 minutes or until soft.
3. Use a sharp knife to mark "X" on the potatoes and fluff pulp with a fork.
4. Top with coconut flakes, chopped apple, Greek yogurt, and maple syrup.
5. Serve immediately.

Nutrition:

Calories: 321

Fat: 3 g

Carbs: 70 g

Protein: 7 g

Sugars: 0.1 g

Sodium: 3%

Flaxseed and Banana Smoothie

Preparation Time: 5 minutes

Cooking Time: 0 minutes

Servings: 4

Ingredients:

- 1 frozen banana
- 1/2 c. almond mil
- Vanilla extract
- 1 tbsp.... almond butter
- 2 tbsp...s. Flaxseed
- 1 tsp.... maple syrup

Directions:

1. Merge all your ingredients to a food processor or blender and run until smooth. Pour the mixture into a glass and enjoy.

Nutrition:

Calories: 376

Fat: 19.4 g

Carbs: 48.3 g

Protein: 9.2 g

Sodium: 64.9 mg

Fruity Tofu Smoothie

Preparation Time: 5 minutes

Cooking Time: 0 minutes

Servings: 2

Ingredients:

- 1 c. ice cold water
- 1 c. packed spinach
- 1/4 c. frozen. mango chunks
- 1/2 c. frozen. pineapple chunks
- 1 tbsp.... chia seeds
- 1 container silken tofu
- 1 frozen. medium banana

Directions:

1. Attach all ingredients in a blender and puree until smooth and creamy.
2. Evenly divide into two glasses, serve and enjoy.

Nutrition:

Calories: 175

Fat: 3.7 g

Carbs: 33.3 g

Protein: 6.0 g

Sugars: 16.3 g

Sodium: 1%

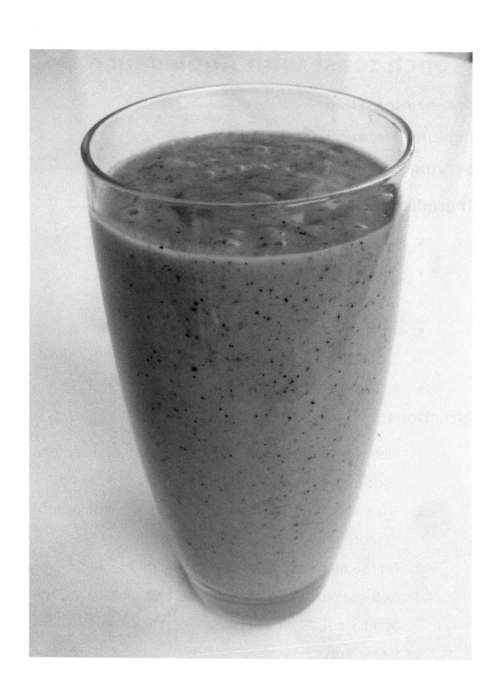

French toast with Applesauce

Preparation Time: 5 minutes

Cooking Time: 5 minutes

Servings: 6

Ingredients:

- 1/4 c. unsweetened applesauce
- 1/2 c. skim milk
- 2 packets Stevia
- 2 eggs
- 6 slices whole wheat bread
- 1 tsp.... ground cinnamon

Directions:

1. Mix well applesauce, sugar, cinnamon, milk and eggs in a mixing bowl.
2. Slice at a time; simmer the bread into applesauce mixture until wet.
3. On medium fire, heat a large nonstick skillet.
4. Add soaked bread on one side and another on the other side.
5. Serve and enjoy.

Nutrition:

Calories: 122.6

Fat: 2.6 g

Carbs: 18.3 g

Protein: 6.5 g

Sugars: 14.8 g

Sodium: 11%

Banana-Peanut Butter 'N Greens Smoothie

Preparation Time: 5 minutes

Cooking Time: 0 minutes

Servings: 1

Ingredients:

- 1 c. chopped and packed Romaine lettuce
- 1 frozen. medium banana
- 1 tbsp.... all-natural peanut butter
- 1 c. cold almond milk

Directions:

1. In a heavy-duty blender, add all ingredients.
2. Puree until smooth and creamy.
3. Serve and enjoy.

Nutrition:

Calories: 349.3

Fat: 9.7 g

Carbs: 57.4 g

Protein: 8.1 g

Sugars: 4.3 g

Sodium: 18%

Baking Powder Biscuits

Preparation Time: 5 minutes

Cooking Time: 5 minutes

Servings: 1

Ingredients:

- 1 egg white
- 1 c. white whole-wheat flour
- 4 tbsp...s. Non-hydrogenated vegetable shortening
- 1 tbsp.... sugar
- 2/3 c. low-
- Fat free milk
- 1 c. unbleached all-purpose flour
- 4 tsp...s. Sodium-free baking powder

Directions:

1. Preheat oven to 450°F.
2. Merge flour, sugar, and baking powder and whip well.
3. Attach the egg white and milk and whip to combine.
4. Set rounds on the baking sheet and bake 10 minutes.
5. Take out the baking sheet and set biscuits on a wire rack to cool.

Nutrition:

Calories: 118,

Fat: 4 g

Carbs: 16 g

Protein: 3 g

Sodium: 6%

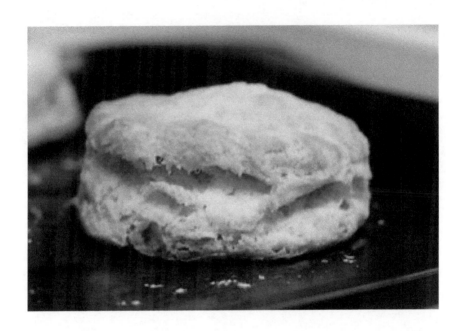

Lunch

Paprika Cauliflower Steaks with Walnut Sauce

Prep time: 5 minutes | Cook time: 30 minutes | Serves 2

Walnut Sauce:

½ cup raw walnut halves

2 tablespoons virgin olive oil, divided

1 clove garlic, chopped

1 small yellow onion, chopped

½ cup unsweetened almond milk

Salt and pepper, to taste

2 tablespoons fresh lemon juice

Paprika Cauliflower:

1 medium head cauliflower

1 teaspoon sweet paprika

1 teaspoon minced fresh thyme leaves (about 2 sprigs)

1. **Preheat the oven to 350ºF (180ºC).**
2. **Make the walnut sauce: Toast the walnuts in a large, ovenproof skillet over medium heat until fragrant and slightly darkened, about 5 minutes. Transfer the walnuts to a blender.**

3. Heat 1 tablespoon of olive oil in the skillet. Add the garlic and onion and sauté for about 2 minutes, or until slightly softened. Transfer the garlic and onion into the blender, along with the almond milk, lemon juice, salt, and pepper. Blend the ingredients until smooth and creamy. Keep the sauce warm while you prepare the cauliflower.

4. Make the paprika cauliflower: Cut two 1-inch-thick "steaks" from the center of the cauliflower. Lightly moisten the steaks with water and season both sides with paprika, thyme, salt, and pepper.

5. Heat the remaining 1 tablespoon of olive oil in the skillet over medium- high heat. Add the cauliflower steaks and sear for about 3 minutes until evenly browned. Flip the cauliflower steaks and transfer the skillet to the oven.

6. Roast in the preheated oven for about 20 minutes until crisp-tender.

7. Serve the cauliflower steaks warm with the walnut sauce on the side.

Per Serving

calories: 367 | fat: 27.9g | protein: 7.0g | carbs: 22.7g | fiber: 5.8g | sodium: 173mg

Potato and Kale Bowls

Prep time: 10 minutes | Cook time: 10 minutes | Serves 4

1 tablespoon olive oil	1½ cups vegetable broth
1 small onion, peeled and diced	2 teaspoons salt
1 stalk celery, diced	½ teaspoon ground black pepper
2 cloves garlic, minced	
4 medium potatoes, peeled and diced	¼ teaspoon caraway seeds
2 bunches kale, washed, deveined, and chopped	1 tablespoon apple cider vinegar
	4 tablespoons sour cream

1. **Press the Sauté button on Instant Pot. Heat oil. Add onion and celery and stir-fry for 3 to 5 minutes until onions are translucent. Add garlic and cook for an additional minute. Add potatoes in an even layer. Add chopped kale in an even layer. Add broth. Lock lid.**

2. **Press the Manual button and adjust time to 5 minutes. Let the pressure release naturally for 10 minutes. Quick release any additional pressure until float valve drops and then unlock lid; then drain broth.**
3. **Stir in salt, pepper, caraway seeds, and vinegar; slightly mash the potatoes in the Instant Pot. Garnish each serving with 1 tablespoon sour cream.**

Per Serving

calories: 259 | fat: 5.5g | protein: 7.9g | carbs: 47.6g | fiber: 7.6g | sodium: 1422mg

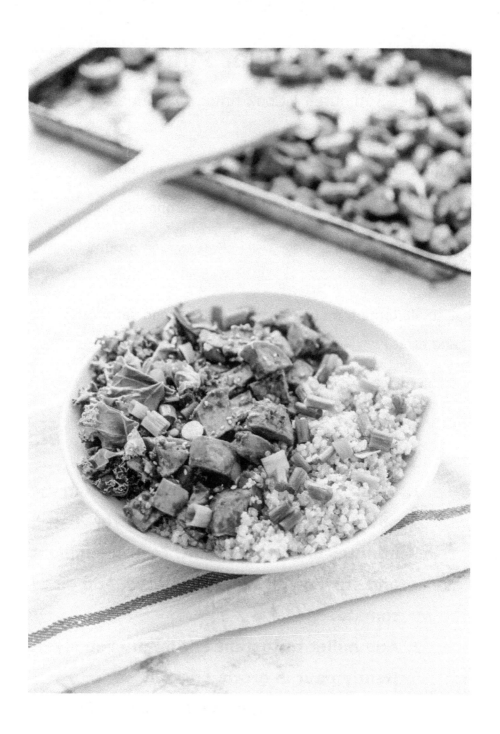

Eggplant and Millet Pilaf

Prep time: 5 minutes | Cook time: 17 minutes | Serves 4

1 tablespoon olive oil

¼ cup peeled and diced onion

1 cup peeled and diced eggplant

1 small Roma tomato, seeded and diced

1 cup millet

2 cups vegetable broth

1 teaspoon sea salt

¼ teaspoon ground black pepper

⅛ teaspoon saffron

⅛ teaspoon cayenne pepper

1 tablespoon chopped fresh chives

1. **Press Sauté button on Instant Pot. Add the olive oil. Add onion and cook for 3 to 5 minutes until translucent. Toss in eggplant and stir-fry for 2 more minutes. Add diced tomato.**
2. **Add millet to Instant Pot in an even layer. Gently pour in broth. Lock lid.**
3. **Press the Rice button (the Instant Pot will determine the time, about 10 minutes**

pressurized cooking time). When timer beeps, let pressure release naturally for 5 minutes. Quick release any additional pressure until float valve drops and then unlock lid.

4. Transfer pot ingredients to a serving bowl. Season with salt, pepper, saffron, and cayenne pepper. Garnish with chives.

Per Serving

calories: 238 | fat: 5.6g | protein: 6.0g | carbs: 40.8g | fiber: 5.3g | sodium: 861mg

Herb Roasted Chicken

Preparation Time: 20 minutes

Cooking Time: 45 minutes

Servings: 2

Ingredients:

- 1 tablespoon virgin olive oil
- 1 whole chicken
- 2 rosemary springs
- 3 garlic cloves (peeled)
- 1 lemon (cut in half)
- 1 teaspoon sea salt
- 1 teaspoon black pepper

Directions:

1. Turn your oven to 450 degrees F.
2. Take your whole chicken and pat it dry using paper towels. Then rub in the olive oil. Remove the leaves from one of the springs of rosemary and scatter them over the chicken. Sprinkle the sea salt and black pepper over top. Place the other whole sprig of rosemary into the cavity of the chicken. Then add in the garlic cloves and lemon halves.
3. Place the chicken into a roasting pan and then place it into the oven. Allow the chicken to bake for 1

hour, then check that the internal temperature should be at least 165 degrees F. If the chicken begins to brown too much, cover it with foil and return it to the oven to finish cooking.

4. When the chicken has cooked to the appropriate temperature remove it from the oven. Let it rest for at least 20 minutes before carving.

5. Serve with a large side of roasted or steamed vegetables or your favorite salad.

Nutrition:

Calories – 309,

Carbs - 1.5 g,

Protein - 27.2 g,

Fat - 21.3 g

Mediterranean bowl

Preparation Time: 25 minutes

Cooking Time: 30 minutes

Servings: 2

Ingredients:

- 2 chicken breasts (chopped into 4 halves)
- 2 diced onions
- 2 bottles of lemon pepper marinade
- 2 diced green bell pepper
- 4 lemon juices
- 8 cloves of crushed garlic.
- 5 teaspoon of olive oil
- Feta cheese
- 1 grape tomato

Directions:

1. 1 large-sized diced zucchini and 1 small-sized. Otherwise, use two medium-sized diced zucchinis.
2. Salt and pepper (according to your desired taste), 4 cups of water.
3. Kalamata olives (as much as you fancy)
4. 1 cup of garbanzo beans

Nutrition:

541 Cal, 34g of protein, 1423mg of potassium, 12g of fiber, 15g of sugar, 72mg of cholesterol, 4g of fat, 45g of carbs.

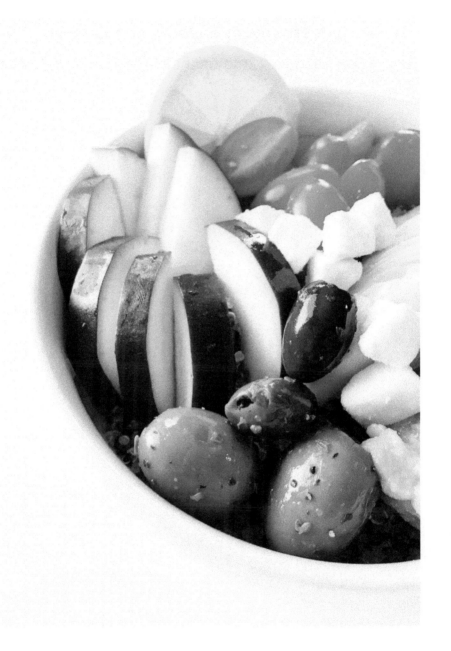

Tasty Lamb Leg

Preparation Time: 10 minutes

Cooking Time: 20 minutes

Servings: 2

Ingredients:

- 2 lbs. leg of lamb, boneless and cut into chunks
- 1 tbsp. olive oil
- 1 tbsp. garlic, sliced
- 1 cup red wine
- 1 cup onion, chopped
- 2 carrots, chopped
- 1 tsp. rosemary, chopped
- 2 tsp. thyme, chopped
- 1 tsp. oregano, chopped
- 1/2 cup beef stock
- 2 tbsp. tomato paste
- Pepper
- Salt

Directions:

1. Add oil into the inner pot of Pressure Pot and set the pot on sauté mode.
2. Add meat and sauté until browned.
3. Add remaining ingredients and stir well.

4. Seal pot with lid and cook on high for 15 minutes.

5. Once done, allow to release pressure naturally. Remove lid.

6. Stir well and serve.

Nutrition:

Calories 540, Fat 20.4 g, Carbohydrates 10.3 g, Sugar 4.2 g, Protein 65.2 g, Cholesterol 204 mg

Kale Sprouts & Lamb

Preparation Time: 10 minutes

Cooking Time: 30 minutes

Servings: 2

Ingredients:

- 2 lbs. lamb, cut into chunks
- 1 tbsp. parsley, chopped
- 2 tbsp. olive oil
- 1 cup kale, chopped
- 1 cup Brussels sprouts, halved
- 1 cup beef stock
- Pepper
- Salt

Directions:

1. Add all ingredients into the inner pot of Pressure Pot and stir well.
2. Seal pot with lid and cook on high for 30 minutes.
3. Once done, allow to release pressure naturally. Remove lid.
4. Serve and enjoy.

Nutrition:

Calories 504,

Fat 23.8 g,

Carbohydrates 3.9 g,

Sugar 0.5 g,

Protein 65.7 g,

Cholesterol 204 mg

Grilled Harissa Chicken

Preparation Time: 20 minutes

Cooking Time: 12 minutes

Servings: 2

Ingredients:

- Juice of 1 lemon
- 1/2 sliced red onion
- 1 ½ teaspoon of coriander
- 1 ½ teaspoon of smoked paprika
- 1 teaspoon of cumin
- 2 teaspoons of cayenne
- Olive oil
- 1 ½ teaspoon of Black pepper
- Kosher salt
- 5 ounces of thawed and drained frozen spinach
- 8 boneless chickens.

Directions:

1. Get a large bowl. Season your chicken with kosher salt on all sides, then add onions, garlic, lemon juice, and harissa paste to the bowl.
2. Add about 3 tablespoons of olive oil to the mixture. Heat a grill to 459 heat (an indoor or outdoor grill works just fine), then oil the grates.

3. Grill each side of the chicken for about 7 minutes. Its temperature should register 165 degrees on a thermometer and it should be fully cooked by then.

Nutrition:

142.5 kcal,

4.7g of fat,

1.2g of saturated fat,

102mg of sodium,

1.7g of carbs,

107.4mg of cholesterol,

22.1g of protein.

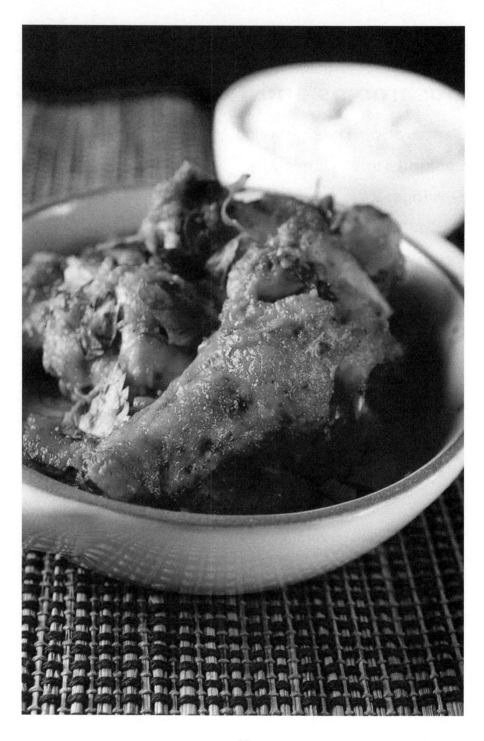

Creamy Rice Risotto with Mushrooms and Thyme

Preparation Time: 20 minutes

Cooking Time: 15 minutes

Servings: 2

Ingredients:

- 2 Tbsp. olive oil
- 1 onion, finely chopped
- 4 garlic cloves, finely chopped
- 13 oz. Arborio rice
- 4 cups sliced mushrooms (use any type!)
- ½ cup dry white wine
- 2 Tbsp. thyme leaves, finely chopped
- 6 ½ cups vegetable or chicken stock
- 3 Tbsp. butter
- ½ cup grated parmesan cheese
- Salt and pepper

Directions:

1. Place the stock into a saucepan over a medium heat, it shouldn't boil, but should be hot and steaming

2. Add the olive oil to a large sauté pan or pot over a medium heat
3. Add the rice and stir to coat in olive oil, allow the rice to become acquainted with the flavor of the onion and garlic, about 3 minutes
4. Add the mushrooms and stir as they soften for about 3 minutes
5. Add zucchinis the onion and garlic and stir as they soften and become fragrant, about 3 minutes the wine and stir to deglaze the corners of the pan, allow it to reduce for about 3 minutes
6. Add the thyme leaves and stir
7. Add a dash of hot stock, stir, and allow it to be absorbed into the rice. Repeat this process, adding dashes of hot stock, stirring, and allowing to absorb, until all of the stock has been used up and the risotto is creamy
8. Stir the butter, parmesan, salt and pepper into the risotto, cover, and leave for at least 5 minutes. This step is crucial for a creamy risotto! The butter and cheese melt, and the starches from the rice have time to relax and create a silky, rich consistency
9. Serve with a little extra sprinkle of grated parmesan and a few thyme leaves!

Nutrition:

Calories: 608; Fat: 19.4 grams; Protein: 23.2 grams; Total carbs: 80.3 grams; Net carbs: 79.8 grams

Pearl Barley, Citrus, and Broccoli Salad

Preparation Time: 25 minutes

Cooking Time: 20 minutes

Servings: 2

Ingredients:

- 1 ½ cups pearl barley
- 4 ¼ cups water
- Salt
- 2 oranges, peeled and chopped
- 1 medium-large head of broccoli, cut into florets
- 3 oz. feta cheese, crumbled
- 1/3 cup chopped almonds, gently toasted
- 1/3 cup chopped hazelnuts, gently toasted
- ½ cup finely chopped parsley
- 3 Tbsp. olive oil
- Salt and pepper

Directions:

1. Place the barley, water, and salt into a saucepan over a medium heat, cover, and bring to boiling point

2. Reduce to a simmer, and partially remove the cover

3. Keep an eye on the barley and add a dash of water if it appears to be drying out

4. When the barley is plump and there is no liquid left, remove the pot from the heat and allow the barley to cool a little

5. Place a steamer over a saucepan of shallow, boiling water, add the broccoli to the steamer, cover, and cook until the broccoli is just cooked but still crunchy and vibrant in color

6. Combine the pearl barley, broccoli, feta, almonds, hazelnuts, parsley, olive oil, salt and pepper in a salad bowl and toss to combine

Nutrition:

Calories: 569, Fat: 28.2 grams, Protein: 19.1 grams, Total carbs: 80 grams, Net carbs: 60 grams

Beetroot and Goat Cheese Salad with Toasted Barley

Preparation Time: 25 minutes

Cooking Time: 15 minutes

Servings: 2

Ingredients:

- 1 ½ cups pearl barley
- 4 ½ cups water
- Salt
- 1 Tbsp. olive oil
- 2 large fresh beets, peeled and cut into chunks
- 1 Tbsp. olive oil
- Fresh thyme
- 4 oz. goat cheese, crumbled
- 6 Tbsp. pumpkin seeds, lightly toasted
- 4 cups baby spinach leaves, roughly chopped
- Salt and pepper
- Juice of 1 lemon

Directions:

1. Preheat the oven to 400 degrees Fahrenheit and line a baking tray with baking paper

2. Lay the beets onto the tray, rub with olive oil, and sprinkle with salt, thyme leaves, and pepper and place into the oven to roast for about 30 minutes or until soft, turning halfway through

3. Place the barley, water, and salt into a saucepan over a medium heat, cover, and bring to boiling point. Reduce the heat and allow the barley to simmer until there's no liquid left, and the barley is chewy

4. Push the beets aside on the baking tray and spread the cooked barley onto the tray and slip into the oven to toast for about 15 minutes (if you're worried about overcooking the beets you can transfer them into a salad bowl at this point)

5. In a salad bowl, toss together the beets, barley, goat cheese, spinach, pumpkin seeds, salt, pepper, and lemon juice.

6. Serve warm or cold

Nutrition:

Calories: 506; Fat: 21.7 grams; Protein: 18.4 grams; Total carbs: 63.8 grams; Net carbs: 50 grams

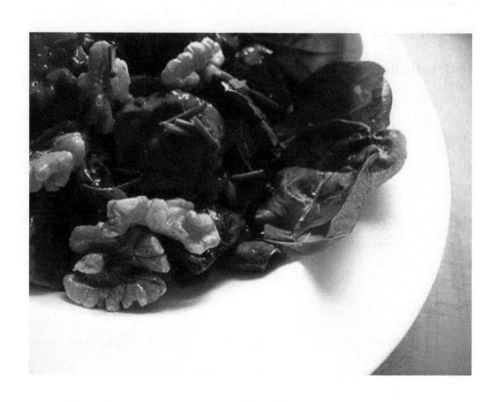

Brown Lentil Salad with Grilled Halloumi

Preparation Time: 15 minutes

Cooking Time: 15 minutes

Servings: 2

Ingredients:

- 2 cans brown lentils (rinsed and drained)
- Juice and zest of 1 lemon
- 2 cups chopped cucumber (I leave the seeds in!)
- ½ cup toasted pine nuts (use almonds or cashews if pine nuts are too expensive in your region)
- 2 Tbsp. olive oil
- 14 oz. halloumi cheese, cut into strips

Directions:

1. Preheat the oven to 450 degrees Fahrenheit and line a baking tray with baking paper
2. In a large salad bowl, toss together the lentils, lemon, cucumber, pine nuts, and olive oil, set aside or refrigerate as you cook the halloumi
3. Place the halloumi slices onto the lined tray and cook in the upper third of the oven for about 12

minutes, turn the slices over, and cook until the other side is golden

4. Serve the salad with halloumi slices on top

Nutrition:

Calories: 665

Fat: 43.7 grams

Protein: 38 grams

Total carbs: 36.7 grams

Net carbs: 27.5 grams

Israeli Couscous with Zucchini, Peas, and Feta

Preparation Time: 15 minutes

Cooking Time: 35 minutes

Servings: 2

Ingredients:

- 2 large zucchinis, cut into rounds
- 2 Tbsp. olive oil
- Salt and pepper
- Rosemary sprig
- 1 lemon, quartered
- 1 Tbsp. olive oil
- 1 Tbsp. butter
- 4 garlic cloves, roughly chopped
- 2 cups Israeli couscous (dry)
- 4 cups chicken or vegetable stock
- Salt and pepper
- 2 cups frozen peas, cooked (microwave, steam, or boil)
- 4 oz. feta cheese, crumbled

Directions:

1. Preheat the oven to 400 degrees Fahrenheit and line a baking tray with baking paper Lay the zucchini rounds onto the tray, rub with olive oil, salt, and pepper. Nestle the rosemary and lemon quarters into the zucchini and slip into the oven to roast for about 30 minutes

2. While the zucchini is cooking, prepare the couscous: add the olive oil, butter, and garlic into a deep-sided sauté pan over a medium heat and allow the butter to melt and become frothy. Add the Israeli couscous, toss in the oil and butter, and toast for about 5 minutes. Add the stock, cover, and leave to cook until the stock has evaporated and the couscous is tender

3. Add the zucchini, peas, and feta to the pan with the couscous. Take the roasted lemon quarters and squeeze the gooey flesh and juices into the couscous and toss to combine

4. Serve warm or cold!

Nutrition: Calories: 610; Fat: 20 grams; Protein: 23.6 grams; Total carbs: 86.5 grams; Net carbs: 76.4 grams

Artichokes Provencal

Preparation Time: 5 minutes

Cooking Time: 15 minutes

Servings: 2

Ingredients:

- 1 Tbsp. olive oil
- 1 onion, roughly chopped
- 4 garlic cloves, finely chopped
- ½ cup dry white wine
- 4 tomatoes, chopped
- 10 oz. artichoke hearts, quartered
- 1 lemon, quartered
- Salt and pepper
- Fresh basil, roughly chopped or torn

Directions:

1. Add the olive oil to a large sauté pan over a medium-high heat
2. Add the onions and garlic and stir as they soften, about 5 minutes
3. Add the wine and allow to reduce for a few minutes
4. Add the artichokes, tomatoes, salt, pepper, and lemon quarters, cover, and cook for about 5-8 minutes or until the artichokes are tender

5. Serve with fresh basil

Nutrition:

Calories: 159

Fat: 7 grams

Protein: 2.8 grams

Total carbs: 15.5 grams

Net carbs: 13.5 grams

Bulgur and Roasted Bell Pepper Salad

Preparation Time: 10 minutes

Cooking Time: 30 minutes

Servings: 2

Ingredients:

- 3 large red bell peppers, seeds removed, sliced
- 1 red onion, sliced
- 2 Tbsp. olive oil
- Salt and pepper
- 2 Tbsp. butter
- 1 Tbsp. olive oil
- 2 cups bulgur (dry)
- 4 cups water
- Salt

Directions:

1. Preheat the oven to 400 degrees Fahrenheit and line a baking tray with baking paper
2. Spread the bell pepper and onion over the tray and rub with olive oil, salt and pepper

3. Roast the bell pepper and onion for about 30 minutes, tossing once, until very soft and slightly charred and gooey

4. Add the butter and oil in a sauté pan over a medium heat

5. When the butter and oil are hot, add the dry bulgur and stir as it toasts, about 2 minutes

6. Add the water and salt to the pan, cover, and cook until the water has evaporated and the bulgur is fluffy and tender

7. Add the roasted bell pepper and onion to the bulgur, toss, and serve

8. Serving suggestions: fresh basil or mint and a side of lemony Greek yogurt

Nutrition:

Calories: 428, Fat: 17 grams, Protein: 10 grams, Total carbs: 63 grams, Net carbs: 51 grams

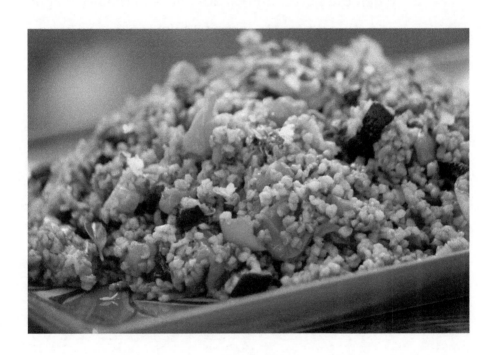

Seafood Stuffing

Preparation Time: 25 minutes

Cooking Time: 30 minutes

Servings: 2

Ingredients:

- 1/2 cup butter
- 1/2 cup chopped green pepper
- 1/2 cup chopped onion
- 1/2 cup chopped celery
- Drained and flaky crabmeat
- 1/2 pound of medium-sized shrimp - peeled and deveined
- 1/2 cup spiced and seasoned breadcrumbs
- 1 mixture of filling for cornbread
- 2 tablespoons of white sugar, divided
- 1 can of mushroom soup (10.75 ounces) condensed
- oz. chicken broth

Directions:

1. Melt the butter in a large frying pan over medium heat. Add pepper, onion, celery crabmeat and shrimp; boil and stir for about 5 minutes. Set aside.
2. In a large bowl, mix stuffing, breadcrumbs, and 1 tablespoon sugar. Stir the vegetables and seafood

63

from the pan. Add the mushroom cream and as much chicken broth as you want. Pour into a 9 x 13-inch baking dish.

3. Bake in the preheated oven for 30 minutes or until lightly roasted.

Nutrition:

344 calories

15.7 grams of fat

28.4 g of carbohydrates

22 g of protein

94 mg of cholesterol

1141 mg of sodium

Scrumptious Salmon Cakes

Preparation Time: 15 minutes

Cooking Time: 15 minutes

Servings: 2

Ingredients:

- 2 cans of salmon, drained and crumbled
- 3/4 cup Italian breadcrumbs
- 1/2 cup chopped fresh parsley
- 2 eggs, beaten
- 2 green onions, minced
- 2 teaspoons seafood herbs
- 1 1/2 teaspoon ground black pepper
- 1 1/2 teaspoons garlic powder
- 3 tablespoons Worcestershire sauce
- 2 tablespoons Dijon mustard
- 3 tablespoons grated Parmesan
- 2 tablespoons creamy vinaigrette
- 1 tablespoon olive oil

Directions:

1. Combine salmon, breadcrumbs, parsley, eggs, green onions, seafood herbs, black pepper, garlic powder, Worcestershire sauce, parmesan cheese,

Dijon mustard, and creamy vinaigrette; divide and shape into eight patties.

2. Heat olive oil in a large frying pan over medium heat. Bake the salmon patties in portions until golden brown, 5 to 7 minutes per side. Repeat if necessary, with more olive oil.

Nutrition:

263 calories, 12.3 g fat, 10.8 g of carbohydrates, 27.8 g of protein, 95 mg cholesterol, 782 mg of sodium

Cajun Seafood Pasta

Preparation Time: 15 minutes

Cooking Time: 16 minutes

Servings: 2

Ingredients:

- 2 cups thick whipped cream
- 1 tablespoon chopped fresh basil
- 1 tablespoon chopped fresh thyme
- 2 teaspoons salt
- 2 teaspoons ground black pepper
- 1 1/2 teaspoon ground red pepper flakes
- 1 teaspoon ground white pepper
- 1 cup chopped green onions
- 1 cup chopped parsley
- 1/2 shrimp, peeled
- 1/2 cup scallops
- 1/2 cup of grated Swiss cheese
- 1/2 cup grated Parmesan cheese
- 1-pound dry fettuccine pasta

Directions:

1. Cook the pasta in a large pot with boiling salted water until al dente.

2. Meanwhile, pour the cream into a large skillet. Cook over medium heat, constantly stirring until it boils. Reduce heat and add spices, salt, pepper, onions, and parsley. Let simmer for 7 to 8 minutes or until thick.

3. Stir seafood and cook until shrimp are no longer transparent. Stir in the cheese and mix well.

4. Drain the pasta. Serve the sauce over the noodles.

Nutrition:

695 calories, 36.7 grams of fat, 62.2 g carbohydrates, 31.5 g of protein, 193 mg cholesterol, 1054 mg of sodium

Seafood Enchiladas

Preparation Time: 15 minutes

Cooking Time: 30 minutes

Servings: 2

Ingredients:

- 1 onion, minced
- 1 tablespoon butter
- 1/2 pound of fresh crab meat
- 1/4-pound shrimp - peeled, gutted and coarsely chopped
- 8 grams of Colby cheese
- 6 flour tortillas (10 inches)
- 1 cup half and half cream
- 1/2 cup sour cream
- 1/4 cup melted butter
- 1 1/2 teaspoon dried parsley
- 1/2 teaspoon garlic salt

Directions:

1. Preheat the oven to 175 ° C (350 ° F).
2. Fry the onions in a large frying pan in 1 tablespoon butter until they are transparent. Remove the pan from the heat and stir in the crab meat and shrimp. Grate the cheese and mix half of the seafood.

3. Place a large spoon of the mixture in each tortilla. Roll the tortillas around the mixture and place them in a 9 x 13-inch baking dish.

4. In a saucepan over medium heat, combine half and half, sour cream, 1/4 cup butter, parsley and garlic salt. Stir until the mixture is lukewarm and mixed. Pour the sauce over the enchiladas and sprinkle with the remaining cheese.

5. Bake in the preheated oven for 30 minutes.

Nutrition:

607 calories, 36.5 grams of fat, 42.6 g carbohydrates, 26.8 g of protein, 136 mg of cholesterol, 1078 mg of sodium

Dinner

Juicy Steak Bites

Preparation Time: 10 minutes

Cooking Time: 9 minutes

Servings: 4

Ingredients:

- 1 lb. sirloin steak, cut into bite-size pieces
- 1 tbsp steak seasoning
- 1 tbsp olive oil
- Pepper
- Salt

Directions:

1. Preheat the air fryer oven to 390 F.
2. Add steak pieces into the large mixing bowl. Add steak seasoning, oil, pepper, and salt over steak pieces and toss until well coated.
3. Transfer steak pieces on air fryer pan and air fry for 5 minutes
4. Turn steak pieces to the other side and cook for 4 minutes more.
5. Serve and enjoy.

Nutrition:

Calories 241

Fat 10.6 g

Carbs 0 g

Protein 34.4 g

Bbq Pork Ribs

Preparation Time: 10 minutes

Cooking Time: 12 minutes

Servings: 6

Ingredients:

- 1 slab baby back pork ribs, cut into pieces
- ½ cup BBQ sauce
- ½ tsp paprika
- Salt

Directions:

1. Add pork ribs in a mixing bowl. Add BBQ sauce, paprika, and salt over pork ribs and coat well and set aside for 30 minutes
2. Preheat the air fryer oven to 350 F. Arrange marinated pork ribs on air fryer oven pan and cook for 10-12 minutes Turn halfway through.
3. Serve and enjoy.

Nutrition:

Calories 145

Fat 7 g

Carbs 10 g

Protein 9 g

Honey Mustard Pork Tenderloin

Preparation Time: 10 minutes

Cooking Time: 26 minutes

Servings: 4

Ingredients:

- 1 lb. pork tenderloin
- 1 tsp sriracha sauce
- 1 tbsp garlic, minced
- 2 tbsp soy sauce
- 1 ½ tbsp honey
- ¾ tbsp Dijon mustard
- 1 tbsp mustard

Directions:

1. Add sriracha sauce, garlic, soy sauce, honey, Dijon mustard, and mustard into the large zip-lock bag and mix well.

2. Add pork tenderloin into the bag. Seal bag and place in the refrigerator for overnight. Preheat the air fryer oven to 380 F. Spray air fryer tray with cooking spray then place marinated pork tenderloin on a tray and air fry for 26 minutes Turn pork tenderloin after every 5 minutes. Slice and serve.

Nutrition:

Calories 195

Fat 4.1 g

Carbs 8 g

Protein 30.5 g

Tomato Corn Risotto

Preparation Time: 10 minutes

Cooking Time: 13 minutes

Servings: 4

Ingredients:

- 1 1/2 cups arborio rice
- 1 cup cherry tomatoes, halved
- 1/4 cup basil, chopped
- 1/4 cup parmesan cheese, grated
- 1/4 cup half and half
- 32 oz vegetable broth
- 1 cup sweet corn
- 3 garlic cloves, minced
- 1/2 cup onion, chopped
- 2 tbsp olive oil
- 4 tbsp butter
- 1 tsp salt

Directions:

1. Add butter into the Pressure Pot and set the pot on sauté mode.
2. Add garlic and onion and sauté for 5 minutes.
3. Add rice and cook for 2-3 minutes.
4. Add broth, corn, pepper, and salt and stir well.

5. Seal pot with lid and cook on high pressure for 6 minutes.

6. Once done then release pressure using the quick-release method than open the lid.

7. Stir in cherry tomatoes, basil, parmesan, and a half and half.

8. Serve and enjoy.

Nutrition:

Calories 548; Fat 24 g; Carbohydrates 69.6 g; Sugar 3.8 g; Protein 14.1 g; Cholesterol 41 mg

Seasoned Pork Tenderloin

Preparation Time: 10 minutes

Cooking Time: 45 minutes

Servings: 5

Ingredients:

- 1½ pounds pork tenderloin
- 2-3 tablespoons BBQ pork seasoning

Directions:

1. Rub the pork with seasoning generously. Insert the rotisserie rod through the pork tenderloin.
2. Insert the rotisserie forks, one on each side of the rod to secure the pork tenderloin.
3. Arrange the drip pan in the bottom of Air Fryer Oven cooking chamber.
4. Select "Roast" and then adjust the temperature to 360 degrees F.
5. Set the timer for 45 minutes and press the "Start".
6. When the display shows "Add Food" press the red lever down and load the left side of the rod into the Air fryer oven.
7. Now, slide the rod's left side into the groove along the metal bar so it doesn't move.

8. Then, close the door and touch "Rotate".

9. Press the red lever to release the rod when cooking time is complete.

10. **Remove the pork from Air fryer oven and place onto a platter for about 10 minutes before slicing.**

11. **With a sharp knife, cut the roast into desired sized slices and serve.**

Nutrition:

Calories 195; Fat 4.8 g; Carbs 0 g; Protein 35.6 g

Roasted Bell Pepper

Preparation Time: 5 minutes

Cooking Time: 20 minutes

Servings: 4

Ingredients:

- 1 Teaspoon Olive Oil
- ½ Teaspoon Thyme
- 4 Cloves Garlic, Minced
- 4 Bell Peppers, Cut into Fourths

Directions:

1. Start by putting your peppers in your air fryer basket and drizzling with olive oil. Make sure they're coated well, and then roast for fifteen minutes.
2. Sprinkle with thyme and garlic, roasting for an additional three to five minutes. They should be tender, and serve warm.

Nutrition:

Calories: 36

Protein: 1 Gram

Fat: 1 Gram

Carbs: 5 Grams

Easy Beef Roast

Preparation Time: 10 minutes

Cooking Time: 45 minutes

Servings: 6

Ingredients:

- 2 ½ lbs. beef roast
- 2 tbsp Italian seasoning

Directions:

1. Arrange roast on the rotisserie spite.
2. Rub roast with Italian seasoning then insert into the air fryer oven.
3. Air fry at 350 F for 45 minutes or until the internal temperature of the roast reaches to 145 F.
4. Slice and serve.

Nutrition:

Calories 365

Fat 13.2 g

Carbs 0.5 g

Protein 57.4 g

Classic Beef Jerky

Preparation Time: 10 minutes

Cooking Time: 4 hours

Servings: 4

Ingredients:

- 2 lbs. London broil, sliced thinly
- 1 tsp onion powder
- 3 tbsp brown sugar
- 3 tbsp soy sauce
- 1 tsp olive oil
- 3/4 tsp garlic powder

Directions:

1. Add all ingredients except meat in the large zip-lock bag.
2. Mix until well combined. Add meat in the bag.
3. Seal bag and massage gently to cover the meat with marinade.
4. Let marinate the meat for 1 hour.
5. Arrange marinated meat slices on air fryer tray and dehydrate at 160 F for 4 hours.

Nutrition:

Calories 133

Fat 4.7 g

Carbs 9.4 g

Protein 13.4 g

Country Style Pork Tenderloin

Preparation Time: 15 minutes

Cooking Time: 25 minutes

Servings: 3

Ingredients:

- 1-pound pork tenderloin
- 1 tablespoon garlic, minced
- 2 tablespoons soy sauce
- 2 tablespoons honey
- 1 tablespoon Dijon mustard
- 1 tablespoon grain mustard
- 1 teaspoon Sriracha sauce

Directions:

1. In a large bowl, add all the ingredients except pork and mix well.
2. Add the pork tenderloin and coat with the mixture generously.
3. Refrigerate to marinate for 2-3 hours.
4. Remove the pork tenderloin from bowl, reserving the marinade.
5. Place the pork tenderloin onto the lightly greased cooking tray.

6. Arrange the drip pan in the bottom of Air Fryer Oven cooking chamber.

7. Select "Air Fry" and then adjust the temperature to 380 degrees F.

8. Set the timer for 25 minutes and press the "Start".

9. When the display shows "Add Food" insert the cooking tray in the center position.

10. **When the display shows "Turn Food" turn the pork and oat with the reserved marinade.**

11. **When cooking time is complete, remove the tray from Air fryer oven and place the pork tenderloin onto a platter for about 10 minutes before slicing.**

12. **With a sharp knife, cut the pork tenderloin into desired sized slices and serve.**

Nutrition:

Calories 277; Fat 5.7 g ; Carbs 14.2 g ; Protein 40.7 g

Glazed Pork Tenderloin

Preparation Time: 15 minutes

Cooking Time: 20 minutes

Servings: 3

Ingredients:

- 1-pound pork tenderloin
- 2 tablespoons Sriracha
- 2 tablespoons honey
- Salt, as required

Directions:

1. Insert the rotisserie rod through the pork tenderloin.
2. Insert the rotisserie forks, one on each side of the rod to secure the pork tenderloin.
3. In a small bowl, add the Sriracha, honey and salt and mix well.
4. Brush the pork tenderloin with honey mixture evenly.
5. Arrange the drip pan in the bottom of Air Fryer Oven cooking chamber.
6. Select "Air Fry" and then adjust the temperature to 350 degrees F.
7. Set the timer for 20 minutes and press the "Start".

8. When the display shows "Add Food" press the red lever down and load the left side of the rod into the Air fryer oven.

9. Now, slide the rod's left side into the groove along the metal bar so it doesn't move.

10. **Then, close the door and touch "Rotate".**

11. **Press the red lever to release the rod when cooking time is complete.**

12. **Remove the pork from Air fryer oven and place onto a platter for about 10 minutes before slicing.**

13. **With a sharp knife, cut the roast into desired sized slices and serve.**

Nutrition:

Calories 269; Fat 5.3 g; Carbs 13.5 g; Protein 39.7 g

Sweet & Spicy Meatballs

Preparation Time: 20 minutes; **Cooking Time:** 30 minutes

Servings: 8

Ingredients:

For Meatballs:

- 2 pounds lean ground beef
- 2/3 cup quick-cooking oats
- ½ cup Ritz crackers, crushed
- 1 (5-ounce) can evaporated milk
- 2 large eggs, beaten lightly
- 1 teaspoon honey
- 1 tablespoon dried onion, minced
- 1 teaspoon garlic powder
- 1 teaspoon ground cumin

For Sauce:

- 1/3 cup orange marmalade
- 1/3 cup honey
- 1/3 cup brown sugar
- 2 tablespoons cornstarch
- 2 tablespoons soy sauce
- 1-2 tablespoons hot sauce
- 1 tablespoon Worcestershire sauce

Directions:

1. For meatballs: in a large bowl, add all the ingredients and mix until well combined.
2. Make 1½-inch balls from the mixture.
3. Arrange half of the meatballs onto a cooking tray in a single layer.
4. Arrange the drip pan in the bottom of Air Fryer Oven cooking chamber.
5. Select "Air Fry" and then adjust the temperature to 380 degrees F.
6. Set the timer for 15 minutes and press the "Start".
7. When the display shows "Add Food" insert the cooking tray in the center position.
8. When the display shows "Turn Food" turn the meatballs.
9. When cooking time is complete, remove the tray from Air fryer oven.
10. **Repeat with the remaining meatballs.**
11. **Meanwhile, for sauce: in a small pan, add all the ingredients over medium heat and cook until thickened, stirring continuously. Serve the meatballs with the topping of sauce.**

Nutrition:

Calories 411; Fat 11.1 g; Carbs 38.8 g; Protein 38.9 g

Herb Butter Rib-Eye Steak

Preparation Time: 10 minutes

Cooking Time: 14 minutes

Servings: 4

Ingredients:

- 2 lbs. rib eye steak, bone-in
- 1 tsp fresh rosemary, chopped
- 1 tsp fresh thyme, chopped
- 1 tsp fresh chives, chopped
- 2 tsp fresh parsley, chopped
- 1 tsp garlic, minced
- ¼ cup butter softened
- Pepper
- Salt

Directions:

1. In a small bowl, combine together butter and herbs.
2. Rub herb butter on rib-eye steak and place it in the refrigerator for 30 minutes
3. Place marinated steak on air fryer oven pan and cook at 400 F for 12-14 minutes
4. Serve and enjoy.

Nutrition:

Calories 416; Fat 36.7 g; Carbs 0.7 g; Protein 20.3 g

Fruits and Desserts

Lemony Tea and Chia Pudding

Prep time: 30 minutes | Cook time: 0 minutes | Serves 3 to 4

2 teaspoons matcha green tea powder (optional)

2 tablespoons ground chia seeds

1 to 2 dates

2 cups unsweetened coconut milk

Zest and juice of 1 lime

1. **Put all the ingredients in a food processor and pulse until creamy and smooth.**
2. **Pour the mixture in a bowl, then wrap in plastic. Store in the refrigerator for at least 20 minutes, then serve chilled.**

Per Serving

calories: 225 | fat: 20.1g | protein: 3.2g | carbs: 5.9g | fiber: 5.0g | sodium: 314mg

Sweet Spiced Pumpkin Pudding

Prep time: 2 hours 10 minutes | Cook time: 0 minutes | Serves 6

1 cup pure pumpkin purée

2 cups unsweetened coconut milk

1 teaspoon ground cinnamon

¼ teaspoon ground nutmeg

½ teaspoon ground ginger

Pinch cloves

¼ cup pure maple syrup

2 tablespoons chopped pecans, for garnish

1. **Combine all the ingredients, except for the chopped pecans, in a large bowl. Stir to mix well.**
2. **Wrap the bowl in plastic and refrigerate for at least 2 hours.**
3. **Remove the bowl from the refrigerator and discard the plastic. Spread the pudding with pecans and serve chilled.**

Per Serving

calories: 249 | fat: 21.1g | protein: 2.8g | carbs: 17.2g | fiber: 3.0g | sodium: 46mg

Mango and Coconut Frozen Pie

Prep time: 1 hour 10 minutes | Cook time: 0 minutes | Serves 8

Crust:

1 cup cashews

½ cup rolled oats

1 cup soft pitted dates

Filling:

2 large mangoes, peeled and chopped

½ cup unsweetened shredded coconut

1 cup unsweetened coconut milk

½ cup water

1. **Combine the ingredients for the crust in a food processor. Pulse to combine well.**
2. **Pour the mixture in an 8-inch springform pan, then press to coat the bottom. Set aside.**
3. **Combine the ingredients for the filling in the food processor, then pulse to purée until smooth.**
4. **Pour the filling over the crust, then use a spatula to spread the filling evenly. Put the pan in the freeze for 30 minutes.**

5. Remove the pan from the freezer and allow to sit for 15 minutes under room temperature before serving.

Per Serving (1 slice)

calories: 426 | fat: 28.2g | protein: 8.1g | carbs: 14.9g | fiber: 6.0g | sodium: 174mg

Mini Nuts and Fruits Crumble

Prep time: 15 minutes | Cook time: 15 minutes | Serves 6

Topping:

¼ cup coarsely chopped hazelnuts

1 cup coarsely chopped walnuts

1 teaspoon ground cinnamon

Sea salt, to taste

1 tablespoon melted coconut oil

Filling:

6 fresh figs, quartered

2 nectarines, pitted and sliced

1 cup fresh blueberries

2 teaspoons lemon zest

½ cup raw honey

1 teaspoon vanilla extract

Make the Topping

1. Combine the ingredients for the topping in a bowl. Stir to mix well. Set aside until ready to use.

Make the Filling:

2. Preheat the oven to 375ºF (190ºC).

3. Combine the ingredients for the fillings in a bowl. Stir to mix well.

4. **Divide the filling in six ramekins, then divide and top with nut topping.**
5. **Bake in the preheated oven for 15 minutes or until the topping is lightly browned and the filling is frothy.**
6. **Serve immediately.**

Per Serving

calories: 336 | fat: 18.8g | protein: 6.3g | carbs: 41.9g | fiber: 6.0g | sodium: 31mg

Cozy Superfood Hot Chocolate

Prep time: 5 minutes | Cook time: 8 minutes | Serves 2

2 cups unsweetened almond milk

1 tablespoon avocado oil

1 tablespoon collagen protein powder

2 teaspoons coconut sugar

2 tablespoons cocoa powder

1 teaspoon ground cinnamon

1 teaspoon ground ginger

1 teaspoon vanilla extract

½ teaspoon ground turmeric

Dash salt

Dash cayenne pepper (optional)

1. In a small saucepan over medium heat, warm the almond milk and avocado oil for about 7 minutes, stirring frequently.
2. Fold in the protein powder, which will only properly dissolve in a heated liquid.
3. Stir in the coconut sugar and cocoa powder until melted and dissolved.
1. Carefully transfer the warm liquid into a blender, along with the cinnamon, ginger,

101

vanilla, turmeric, salt, and cayenne pepper (if desired). Blend for 15 seconds until frothy.

4. Serve immediately.

Per Serving

calories: 217 | fat: 11.0g | protein: 11.2g | carbs: 14.8g | fiber: 6.0g | sodium: 202mg

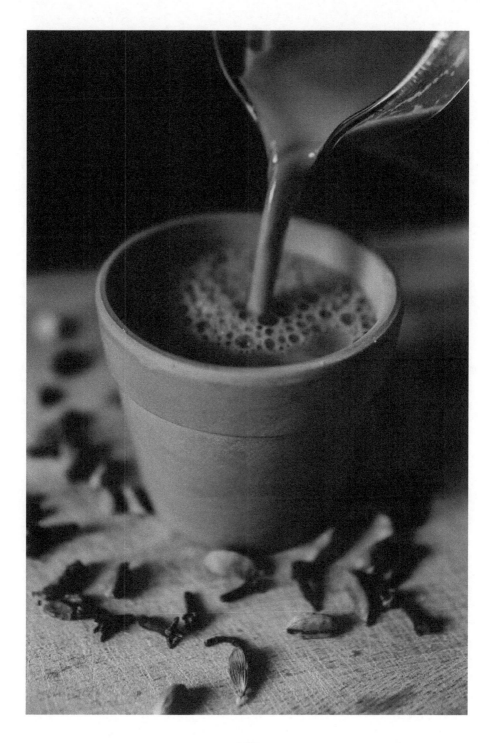

Quinoa Bake with Banana

Preparation Time: 15 minutes

Cooking Time: 1 hour & 10 minutes

Servings: 8

Ingredients:

- 3 cups medium over-ripe Bananas, mashed
- 1/4 cup molasses
- 1/4 cup pure maple syrup
- 1 tbsp cinnamon
- 2 tsp raw vanilla extract
- 1 tsp ground ginger
- 1 tsp ground cloves
- 1/2 tsp ground allspice
- 1/2 tsp salt
- 1 cup quinoa, uncooked
- 2 1/2 cups unsweetened vanilla almond milk
- 1/4 cup slivered almonds

Directions:

1. In the bottom of a 2 1/2-3-quart casserole dish, mix together the mashed banana, maple syrup, cinnamon, vanilla extract, ginger, cloves, allspice, molasses, and salt until well mixed.

2. Add in the quinoa, stir until the quinoa is evenly in the banana mixture. Whisk in the almond milk, mix until well combined, cover and refrigerate overnight or bake immediately.

3. Heat oven to 350 degrees F. Whisk the quinoa mixture making sure it doesn't settle to the bottom.

4. Cover the pan with tinfoil and bake until the liquid is absorbed, and the top of the quinoa is set, about 1 hour to 1 hour and 15 minutes.

5. Turn the oven to high broil, uncover the pan, sprinkle with sliced almonds, and lightly press them into the quinoa.

6. Broil until the almonds just turn golden brown, about 2-4 minutes, watching closely, as they burn quickly. Allow to cool for 10 minutes then slice the quinoa bake

7. Distribute the quinoa bake among the containers, store in the fridge for 3-4 days.

Nutrition:

Calories:213; Carbs: 41g; Fat: 4g; Protein: 5g

Feta Cheesecake

Preparation Time: 30 Minutes

Cooking Time: 90 Minutes

Servings: 12

Ingredients:

- 2 cups graham cracker crumbs (about 30 crackers)
- ½ tsp ground cinnamon
- 6 tbsps. unsalted butter, melted
- ½ cup sesame seeds, toasted
- 12 ounces cream cheese, softened
- 1 cup crumbled feta cheese
- 3 large eggs
- 1 cup of sugar
- 2 cups plain yogurt
- 2 tbsps. grated lemon zest
- 1 tsp vanilla

Directions:

1. Set the oven to 350°F.
2. Mix the cracker crumbs, butter, cinnamon, and sesame seeds with a fork. Move the combination to a springform pan and spread until it is even. Refrigerate.

3. In a separate bowl, mix the cream cheese and feta. With an electric mixer, beat both kinds of cheese together. Add the eggs one after the other, beating the mixture with each new addition. Add sugar, then keep beating until creamy. Mix in yogurt, vanilla, and lemon zest.

4. Bring out the refrigerated springform and spread the batter on it. Then place it in a baking pan. Pour water in the pan till it is halfway full.

5. Bake for about 50 minutes. Remove cheesecake and allow it to cool. Refrigerate for at least 4 hours.

6. It is done. Serve when ready.

Nutrition:

Calories: 98kcal; Carbs: 7g; Fat: 7g; Protein: 3g

Pear Croustade

Preparation Time: 30 Minutes

Cooking Time: 60 Minutes

Servings: 10

Ingredients:

- 1 cup plus 1 tbsp. all-purpose flour, divided
- 4 ½ tbsps. Sugar, divided
- 1/8 tsp salt
- 6 tbsps. Unsalted butter, chilled, cut into ½ inch cubes
- 1 large-sized egg, separated
- 1 ½ tbsps. Ice-cold water
- 3 firm, ripe pears (Bosc), peeled, cored, sliced into ¼ inch slices 1 tbsp. fresh lemon juice
- 1/3 tsp ground allspice
- 1 tsp anise seeds

Directions:

1. Pour 1 cup of flour, 1 ½ Tbsps. Of sugar, butter, and salt into a food processor and combine the ingredients by pulsing.
2. Whisk the yolk of the egg and ice water in a separate bowl. Mix the egg mixture with the flour

mixture. It will form a dough, wrap it, and set aside for an hour.

3. Set the oven to 400°F.
4. Mix the pear, sugar, leftover flour, allspice, anise seed, and lemon juice in a large bowl to make a filling.
5. Arrange the filling on the center of the dough.
6. Bake for about 40 minutes. Cool for about 15 minutes before serving.

Nutrition:

Calories: 498kcal

Carbs: 32g

Fat: 32g

Protein: 18g

Lightning Source UK Ltd.
Milton Keynes UK
UKHW021014240621
386072UK00001B/50